COMPLEMENTARY AND ALTERNATIVE MEDICINE AMONG CHINESE CANADIANS

PUBLIC HEALTH IN THE 21ST CENTURY

Additional books in this series can be found on Nova's website
under the Series tab.

Additional E-books in this series can be found on Nova's website
under the E-books tab.

COMPLEMENTARY AND ALTERNATIVE MEDICINE AMONG CHINESE CANADIANS

MARILYN A. ROTH

AND

KAREN M. KOBAYASHI

Nova Biomedical
Nova Science Publishers, Inc.
New York

For permission to use material from this book please contact us:
Telephone 631-231-7269; Fax 631-231-8175
Web Site: http://www.novapublishers.com

Library of Congress Cataloging-in-Publication Data

ISBN: 978-1-61728-014-6

Published by Nova Science Publishers, Inc. ✛ *New York*

Contents

Preface

This book examines the relationship between Chinese Canadian ethnicity and the use of complementary and alternative medicine (CAM) and explores some of the factors that contribute to CAM use among this visible minority group. Using data from the 2003 Canadian Community Health Survey, we employ multivariate logistic regression techniques to investigate the extent to which CAM use varies among Chinese Canadians and non-Chinese Canadians. Two three-way interactions, which demonstrate how the combination of certain identity markers increases their predictive value within the model, are also examined. The results indicate that use of complementary and alternative medicine varies according to ethnicity, with Chinese Canadians being more likely to use than non-Chinese Canadians. Further, we find that cultural factors play a key role in establishing the necessary conditions for increasing the likelihood of CAM use for Chinese Canadians. Indeed, two of the three most commonly sought CAM modalities (i.e., acupuncture and herbal medicine) used by Chinese Canadians are rooted in Traditional Chinese Medicine (TCM), thereby implicating cultural markers in CAM use. Other important factors that are found to facilitate CAM use among the Chinese include *social capital*, as indicated by sense of belonging to local community, the cultural context of their community, and the extent to which their place of residence is *institutionally complete*. Findings are discussed in terms of their implications for health care policy and program development for visible minority immigrant adults.

Chapter I

Introduction

Recent studies on health care utilization have reported that an increasing number of Canadians and Americans are using complementary and alternative medicine (CAM) (Barnes, Bloom, & Nahin, 2007; Bodeker & Kronenberg, 2002; Suzuki, 2004; Boon, Verhoef, Vanderheyden, & Westlake, 2006; Eisenberg, Kessler, Foster, Norlock, Calkins, & Delbanco, 1993; Eisenberg, Davis, Ettner, Appel, Wilkey, Van Rompay, and Kessler, 1998). It has been reported that as many as 42% of Americans and at least 15% of Canadians regularly use some type of CAM (Eisenberg et al., 1998; Millar, 1997), and members of visible minority groups like the Chinese, for whom CAM use is prevalent (Mackenzie, Taylor, Bloom, Hufford, & Johnson, 2003), often utilize a combination of CAM practitioners and conventional medical doctors, (Pourat, Lubben, Wallace, & Moon, 1999; Mackenzie et al., 2003). This is not surprising since most CAM practices are rooted in visible minority cultures (e.g., acupuncture is rooted in traditional Chinese medicine, yoga has origins in Ayurvedic medicine, and herbal remedies are rooted in Chinese, Ayurvedic, and other traditional Asian forms of medicine); that is, many such practices are consistent with the traditional customs and beliefs of visible minorities, particularly the foreign-born (Hufford, 2002; Mackenzie et al., 2003).

Canada has welcomed, on average, more than 200,000 new immigrants each year since 1990, with more than one million arriving between 2001 and 2006 (Statistics Canada, 2008), resulting in a changing demographic landscape. Between 2001 and 2006, Canada's foreign-born population grew by 13.6%, while the Canadian-born population grew by only 3.3% (Statistics Canada, 2008). The Mainland Chinese had been the largest incoming group each year since 1998; however, according to the most recent iteration of the

Census from 2006, the South Asians have now overtaken the Chinese. Including immigrants from Hong Kong and Taiwan, the Chinese have been one of the two largest groups for over ten years (Statistics Canada, 2008).

Some researchers attribute part of the increase in CAM use to this emergent ethnocultural diversity given the roots of CAM practices in visible minority health care traditions (Hufford, 2002; Mackenzie et al., 2003). In addition, cultural and structural barriers exist that affect immigrants' access to treatment and/or tests through the Canadian health care system (Kobayashi, 2003). Given access issues and the familiarity of CAM practices from their home countries then, it is not surprising that many visible minority immigrants may feel more comfortable and, thus, be more likely to use CAM practices to treat illness and/or maintain their health. Consequently, it is essential that governments address the congruence (or lack thereof) between the services visible minority Canadians need and the services the existing health care system provides.

It is important to consider patients' "culturally developed world views" in order to understand how they learn and think about their own health (Kakai, Maskarinec, Shumay, Tatsumura, & Tasaki, 2003:851). In the case of CAM use, immigrant status, time since immigration, and ethnicity are important factors in providing insight into the health care treatments people choose (Bair, Gale, Greendale, Sternfeld, Adler, Azari, & Harkey, 2002; Kakai et al., 2003; Hufford, 1995). In turn, recognizing the factors influencing this selection process is important for improving the delivery of care (Pourat et al., 1999). Knowing the types of care people prefer may help to improve the efficiency and effectiveness of the overall system and its ability to provide care by addressing, or at least becoming more sensitive to, certain barriers to access related to cultural traditions and beliefs beyond just language. Indeed, although research indicates that people are shaped by their culture and ethnicity, which, in turn, influence their actions and decisions (Nagel, 1994), it is important to establish whether these factors continue to influence immigrants after migration and settlement. And, if so, it is important to understand why members of certain largely immigrant groups, such as the Chinese, decide to continue using alternative health practices post-immigration.

"Situating" CAM

The topic being covered in this book   is situated in the context of a broader social issue: the continuing power imbalances and hierarchical systems that perpetuate inequality by locating CAM as an "othered" set of practices, while simultaneously devaluing the health beliefs[2] of immigrants and visible minorities like the Chinese. Despite the fact that traditional Chinese medical practices were established in China centuries ago, continued use of traditional health practices upon arrival to Canada may actually serve to further marginalize Chinese Canadians. When differences are not openly acknowledged, Chinese Canadians who adhere to these practices may feel insecure (Fink, 2002). Consequently, some would argue that the existing health care system with its emphasis on universal access is inadequate because it fails to meet the needs of many Chinese Canadians, both foreign and Canadian-born. Because the dominance of the biomedical model is at the core of this system, it could be argued that the system needs to be refined so as to allow all Canadians the freedom to choose which type of health care services are most appropriate to meet their needs. There is a need then for policymakers to confront the long-standing inequality within the health care system stemming from biomedicine's historic monopoly over health care and treatment (Saks, 2000).

This book examines the relationship between Chinese Canadian ethnicity and the use of complementary and alternative medicine in Canada, and explores some of the factors that contribute to CAM use among this visible minority group. Using secondary data analysis, this study: (1) examines the extent to which CAM use varies among Chinese Canadians and non-Chinese Canadians (by immigrant status, charter language ability, socio-economic status, gender, and other diversity markers); and (2) provides insights into the reasons why Chinese Canadians use CAM. In this study CAM use is defined as having used at least one form of unconventional health care (e.g., herbal medicine, acupuncture, massage therapy) during the past year. This is consistent with the definition used in the Canadian Community Health Survey (CCHS). We recognize that this definition is limited by its inability to address major issues, such as power, mandate, and regulation, that exist between CAM practices. It is important to acknowledge, therefore, the diversity that exists within CAM and recognize that a single mandate or type of regulation is not suitable for all CAM practices because of these vast differences. It is also important to acknowledge that this diversity among CAM practices also translates into power differentials across practices within the field of alternative medicine. In addition, in this chapter Chinese Canadian is also

---

[2] Good (1994) argues that the term *health beliefs* is problematic based on how the meaning of the word 'belief' has evolved. With this in mind, in this book *health beliefs* should be conceptualized as the way in which people understand health and illness.

defined based on the CCHS, which includes people who self-identify as being of Chinese ethnic origin or a combination of Chinese and other ethnic origins. This includes people born in Mainland China, Taiwan, Hong Kong, Macao, Canada, and numerous other countries. This operationalization has limitations in that the definition of Chinese Canadian should be based on more than country of birth. Indeed, of importance here is an acknowledgement that the Chinese Canadian population is diverse in that there are cultural and linguistic (including dialectic) differences between these groups which can shape understandings of health and illness, which, in turn, can affect patterns of CAM utilization. Because of limited sample sizes for some of these groups, however, all Chinese Canadians have been grouped together for purposes of the analysis.

Some of the factors that may contribute to CAM use among Chinese Canadians that are examined include: alternative/traditional health ideologies and beliefs; immigrant status; region of birth/residence prior to immigration; time since immigration; the nature and number of chronic condition(s); discontent with conventional medicine and the extent to which the geographic community of residence is *institutionally complete* (see Astin, 1998; Mackenzie et al., 2003; Millar, 1997; Najm et al., 2003; Struthers & Nichols, 2004; Lee et al., 2001).

While some Canadian literature regarding CAM use exists (McFarland, Bigelow, Zani, Newsom, & Kaplan, 2002; Millar, 1997), there has been very little research that examines the relationship between immigrant status, ethnicity (particularly Chinese), and CAM use. Focusing on Chinese Canadians is particularly relevant since they are the second largest visible minority group in Canada, with nearly 75% being foreign-born. Chinese Canadians comprise 3.9% of Canada's total population, which translates into more than one million people. Ontario's population is over 4% Chinese Canadian, while Metropolitan Toronto is almost 10% Chinese. Chinese Canadians comprise 10% of British Columbia's population, and over 18% of Metropolitan Vancouver's population (Statistics Canada, 2008).

CAM use among Canada's Chinese population is a salient health care policy issue within the context of re-defining the Canadian health care system and the delivery of culturally sensitive care to all Canadians. This book assists in guiding policy development by providing policymakers with population health-based knowledge about the extent to which Chinese Canadians are using CAM, as well as much-needed insight into the reasons for its use.

Chapter II

Conceptual Framework

The concept of *institutional completeness* refers to the social organization of ethnic communities and the extent to which these communities can provide all the services that are required by its members (Breton, 1964; Hedley, 1980). The cultural context of a community, which is partly determined by the extent to which the community is *institutionally complete*, may affect the lifestyle choices its members make, as well as the activities and even health care practices in which they participate. Thus, the extent to which a community is *institutionally complete* may help to predict whether or not traditional cultural ideologies and practices will be prevalent and maintained within that community.

There are numerous Chinese communities in Toronto and Vancouver that have achieved some level of *institutional completeness*. As a result, the Chinese in these communities have greater "resources" or *cultural capital* to maintain support for "subgroup activities and institutions" through, among other things, the accumulation of *social capital* (Fong & Wilkes, 2003). The term *social capital* is generally used to acknowledge the resources that are amassed through social relations (Bourdieu, 1997). The concept can be used to explicate how social relations and common values influence attitudes and behaviours, in addition to providing insight into how relationships, communities, and socio-environmental factors may aid in understanding the health-seeking behaviours of different populations. *Social capital* coupled with *institutional completeness* facilitates commonality between community members with respect to the beliefs they hold and the services they use (Breton, 1964; Hedley, 1980; White, Fong, & Cai, 2003). *Institutional completeness* and *social capital* are very much linked to the processes of acculturation and assimilation that immigrants undergo following their arrival to a host country. The study that is central to this book allows us to gather insights into how living in a partially *institutionally complete* community and how high levels of *social capital* may impact the CAM utilization patterns of Chinese Canadians.

Chapter III

What Is Health? Definitions and Viewpoints from Biomedicine and CAM

The World Health Organization (WHO) defines health as "a state of complete physical, mental, and social well-being and not merely the absence of disease or infirmity" (WHO, 2010). Contrary to biomedicine's definition, the WHO's definition of health encompasses a more holistic perspective, which recognizes the importance of mental, physical, and social health and well-being. The biomedical model largely fails to encompass non-biological factors as contributors to health and well-being. While specific CAM practices may only consider some of these factors implicitly, the general, underlying philosophy and framework of most practices allow for all of these aspects to be considered (either explicitly or implicitly) when treating a person (Bates, 2000). Despite the seemingly radical differences between biomedicine and CAM, the very use of the term "complementary" implies at least some level of compatibility between the two systems. Thus, rather than conceiving biomedicine and CAM as opposites, it is more appropriate to conceptualize their underlying philosophies regarding health care along a continuum, whereby different facets of each system fall at different places along a continuum. With this in mind, further inquiry into both approaches is essential in order to understand why the standard biomedical definition of health, which emphasizes curative treatments rather than preventative health maintenance, is insufficient. This is important given that many forms of CAM emphasize preventative health care, a subject that deserves more attention within

Canada's biomedically-dominated health care system. It should be noted that since CAM is often operationalized in opposition to biomedicine within the literature, the following examination of biomedicine is limited. Biomedicine's definition of health fails to recognize the systems using this notion that their approaches are best conceptualized along a continuum rather than as a dichotomy.

Canada's existing health care system is based primarily on the framework of biomedicine (Mishler, 1981). The biomedical model is entrenched within the Canadian system, viewing health as the absence of disease and focusing almost entirely on the biological determinants of disease and illness. This framework has four main assumptions: (1) disease represents "deviations from normal functioning," (2) the doctrine of specific etiology, (3) the assumption of generic diseases, and (4) the scientific neutrality of medicine (Mishler, 1981). As a result, the health care system has focused primarily on acute care, which in turn, often only provides temporary solutions without solving underlying problems (McKinlay, 1994). In addition to being almost exclusively focused on "cure" rather than prevention, another major shortcoming of the biomedical framework is that, for the most part, it fails to consider the social context in which illness is experienced. Consequently, the model is limited in its ability to address health issues across different cultures (Helman, 1991). Although biological components are an important part of medicine, illness is much more complex than these components alone.

Granted, over the past few decades Canada's health care system has acknowledged the importance of some aspects of the population health model which, despite being based on the biomedical model, considers many social determinants of health, including factors such as hierarchy, social status, and social cohesion, in addition to demographic characteristics like age, gender, income, education, and ethnicity (Evans, 1994; Muntaner, Lynch, & Oates, 2002; McDonough & Walters, 2001). However, according to Evans and Stoddart (1994), even though social determinants of health included in the population health model have been acknowledged and recognized as important, both the federal and provincial governments have largely failed to create and implement policy that deals with the inequalities people experience, a failure that has resulted in the perpetuation of negative effects on health. Even though evidence from research addressing topics like environmental sanitation, quality of nutrition and shelter, stress, and social environment clearly points to a relationship between social inequalities and poor health, the government has not directly addressed these problems through its health care policies and/or programs (Evans & Stoddart, 1994).

Inhorn and Whittle (2001) argue that some health models perpetuate social inequalities in health even though they were developed to alleviate such disparities. This is linked to Conrad's (1992) evaluation of medicalization as a form of social control, which can operate through dominant ideology (i.e. biomedical knowledge) and practice (i.e. services covered under Medicare). To change this, the system requires a renewed focus on the "upstream" which may ultimately require a fundamental change in Canada's underlying political ideology, with the government taking more responsibility for the overall well-being of its people (McKinlay, 1994; Navarro & Shi, 2001).

Unlike the biomedical model, CAM approaches illness and disease in a more holistic way, taking body and mind into consideration. Thus, one possible place to begin changing the system is with CAM, which focuses on the overall well-being of individuals, including their social, cultural, and often spiritual identities, in the treatment of illness. In fact, Struthers and Nichols (2004) suggest that CAM is used or at least could be used to reduce inequality with regard to health and health care among marginalized people, including immigrants and visible minorities, because CAM practices often provide a more culturally appropriate style of health care. CAM may also help alleviate some of the barriers to access that immigrants often face if traditional ways of treating illness could be delivered by practitioners who have similar ways of understanding health and illness, who use familiar terminology, and who may even speak the same language. Using CAM to help reduce inequality and alleviate barriers to access is consistent with a relatively new initiative in health care delivery called "mainstreaming," which works to make health care services more accessible to visible minority Canadians (Hudspith, 2005).

The debate between "mainstreaming" and "dedicated programs and services" is especially relevant considering Canada's visible minority population has and continues to increase substantially. While "mainstreaming" aims to acknowledge and include ethnicity and culture as important elements to consider when making policy or planning services, "dedicated programs and services" are developed for specific ethnocultural groups (Hudspith, 2005). The implementation of "dedicated programs and services" is problematic in that these programs and services facilitate segregation, which may lead to further misunderstanding and intolerance. On the other hand, "mainstreaming" values cultural diversity and allows for culturally sensitive care while, at the same time, promoting integration into Canadian society by establishing an underlying set of common values (in this case, relating to health care) that, ideally, everyone accepts. Ultimately, the promotion of integration, inclusion, and solidarity rather than segregation, exclusion, and discord are better attained using a "mainstreaming" approach, which is also more consistent with the basic tenets of Canada's Multiculturalism Act (Department of Justice Canada, 2010). In the context of health care then, one way to make services more culturally sensitive is to make CAM available to all Canadians. A more thorough discussion of CAM will provide insights into why certain visible minority groups may want access to these services.

Chapter IV

What is CAM?

A working definition of CAM is needed here to provide an understanding of how its approach to health differs from that of the biomedical model. CAM consists of a diverse group of perspectives and approaches to health, which are supported by a variety of theories, observations, facts, values, and social elements (Hufford, 2002). CAM includes many forms of care, such as naturopathy, chiropractic, homeopathy, herbal remedies, acupuncture and other traditional Chinese medicine, midwifery, and Ayurvedic medicine, in addition to more self-administered, less formal types of care, such as folk medicine. Different forms of CAM have varying levels of acceptance within mainstream Canadian society. Some modalities, like chiropractors and midwives, have governing bodies, professional organizations, and mandates, and their practitioners are regulated and licensed. Therefore, degrees of power range among CAM modalities within the field of alternative health care; this is in addition to the power imbalance that exists between CAM and biomedicine within the broader field of health care in Canada. CAM practices that may be viewed as having more power (i.e., chiropractors, massage therapists, and midwives) are often the modalities that have sought or are seeking professionalization through regulation and licensing. Moreover, the steady increase in the utilization of CAM could be perceived as a social movement, but this social movement may be limited to certain forms of CAM that have been deemed more "legitimate" because they have professional organizations and mandates, some level of state support (i.e., through insurance), and have developed a loyal, more educated client following. Other forms of CAM that lack regulation and therefore legitimation like TCM or Ayurvedic medicine may be perceived as being a fringe or alternative social movement due to the "average" demographic profile of their clientele (i.e., visible minority, immigrant, less educated), which may, in turn, link practices like TCM to culturally "different" (i.e., traditional ethnic immigrant) understandings of health.

The Canadian College of Naturopathic Medicine (CCNM) defines naturopathic medicine, which incorporates many forms of alternative medicine, as "a complete and coordinated approach to health care" which includes "diagnosis, treatment, and prevention using natural therapies and gentle techniques… integrating scientific knowledge with traditional healing wisdom" (CCNM, 2010). Like some aspects of conventional medicine, what underlies all forms of CAM is a strong emphasis on removing the causes of illness rather than just the symptoms. In addition, consistent with the WHO's definition of health, CAM recognizes that physical, mental, emotional, genetic, environmental, and social factors all contribute to a person's health status (CCNM, 2010). Alternative medicine's overarching ideology recognizes that a myriad of factors can affect a person's health and may, in fact, be manifested through specific symptoms or illnesses, and that each of these factors is important when treating patients. CAM requires that a person maintain a balance of body and soul to be considered healthy, but biomedicine only considers the body and reduces it to different parts rather than viewing it as a functioning whole. The biomedical model also fails to identify and define what constitutes "normal," an often vague and undefined term in the context of health.

Chapter V

Trends in CAM Use

Despite the existence of a diversity of health care practices and beliefs, Canadian health culture over the past century has been limited to allopathic medicine, acknowledging this model as its convention. Conventional medicine has largely treated CAM in a very paternalistic fashion, often questioning and trying to discredit CAM practices so as to further its own objectives. In fact, up until the 1980s, alternative medicine use was often associated with low income and low education as well as ethnic and religious minorities. Many believed that CAM practices would no longer be desirable and would eventually disappear as people became better educated and biomedicine became increasingly accessible to all (Hufford, 2002).

Despite biomedicine's "medicocentric" claims and its attempt to restrict health care to practices within the boundaries of conventional medicine, CAM has continued to grow in popularity, especially over the past 15 years (Hufford, 2002:30). A 2001 Health Canada publication reported that 25% of Canadians regularly use some form of CAM. According to a 1994-1995 study by Millar (1997), this proportion is more conservatively estimated at 15% of Canadians over 15 years of age. Regardless of the exact percentage, researchers agree that general use of CAM is on the rise (Suzuki, 2004; Astin, 1998; Eisenberg et al., 1993). CAM and other "traditional" forms of medicine are not only popular in Canada, they are common all around the world, with 42% of Americans, 48% of Australians, 49% of the French, 40% of Chinese, and almost 80% of Africans regularly using traditional and/or CAM (Bodeker & Kronenberg, 2002). However, as stated earlier, the methods and definitions used to collect these statistics were probably not standardized, and should be interpreted with caution. Despite this methodological issue, these figures point to a general interest and, in Western countries, an increase in the utilization of CAM practices over time. In Canada, CAM use has been found to be most common among women, older adults between the ages of 45 and 64, people with higher education and incomes, and those suffering from at least one form of chronic illness (Millar, 1997).

While most studies to date have focused on who uses alternative medicine, a few studies have attempted to understand why people choose to use CAM (see Astin, 1998; Kelner and Wellman, 1997). To date, however, there have been even fewer studies that have focused on ethnocultural minorities' reasons for use. These studies generally conclude that the decision to use CAM is based on a combination of factors, such as being discontented with conventional medicine, having an "alternative ideology," trusting public and private testimonials regarding CAM's effectiveness, and being in tune with a variety of different social movements (Astin, 1998; Kelner and Wellman, 1997:209; Furnham and Vincent, 2000). Kelner and Wellman (1997) used the Anderson Socio-behavioural model to examine the factors that influence why people use CAM. This model examines how *predisposing* factors, such as age and education, *enabling* factors, including community and personal resources that make CAM accessible, and the *need* for care, such as suffering from a chronic illness, influence people's decisions to use CAM. According to their findings, there is clearly a relationship between social, structural, and health variables that predisposes people to CAM use. Kelner and Wellman (1997) describe those who hold an "alternative ideology" or alternative health beliefs as being more committed to preventative health care (which is connected to a personal emphasis on health maintenance), having a more holistic view of health, being more open to alternative therapies, and wanting more personal control over their health and health-related decisions.

Chapter VI

Ethnicity and Health Care Choices: Ethnic Enclaves, Institutional Completeness, Social Capital, and Acculturation

Culture is often associated with ethnicity, and for members of ethnocultural minority groups, their identities create collective meaning and community and serve as a basis for mobilization (Alund, 2003). It is through the construction of identity based on ethnicity and culture that visible minorities may confront problems and make decisions (Nagel, 1994). It is apparent that medicine and health beliefs are culturally constructed because different types of health care and health ideologies are produced by different cultures (Mckenzie et al., 2003). For example, TCM was developed by the Chinese, Ayurvedic medicine by South Asians, and homeopathy by the Germans, while the tenets of Western biomedicine are rooted in ancient Greek culture.

It is curious that biomedicine largely monopolizes insured health care in North America, despite the fact that many people's health beliefs are not necessarily congruent with the biomedical model (Mckenzie et al., 2003). Indeed, many people subscribe to different health beliefs, the majority of whom are immigrants and visible minorities. Given that an individual's identity is greatly shaped by ethnicity and other cultural factors, such influences may have a significant impact on the formation of his/her attitudes, decisions, and actions with regards to physical and mental health (Nagel, 1994; Hufford, 2002).

The cultural context of the lives of visible minorities, regardless of immigrant status, influences their decisions and willingness to adhere to certain ideologies and practices. This includes their decisions and actions regarding health and health care. The size and strength of an ethnic community in addition to the number of services it provides is directly related to its ability to impose (and maintain) dominant cultural ideologies and practices onto individuals (Breton, 1964; Hedley, 1980; White, Fong, & Cai, 2003). As was discussed previously, research in this area has focused primarily on the establishment of ethnic enclaves and the extent to which these communities are *institutionally complete* (see White et al., 2003; Fong & Wilkes, 2003; Fennema; 2004). It can be expected that visible minority immigrants who live in ethnic enclaves that have multiple elements of *institutional completeness* would be more likely to adhere to traditional health practices and beliefs than those who live in other "less complete" communities.

The majority of visible minority immigrants typically settle in one of Canada's three largest cities: Toronto, Montreal, and Vancouver (Fong & Wilkes, 2003). These cities have well-established visible minority communities, which include ethnic neighbourhoods and residential spaces. The term 'ethnic enclave' usually refers to communities that consist of immigrants who have voluntarily chosen to cluster together in a neighborhood. While places of residence are important within ethnic enclaves, enclaves are sustained by locally run businesses (Wilson & Portes, 1980). Large cities typically have segregated residential patterns based on ethnic and cultural distinctions, including language, customs, and institutions (Fong & Wilkes, 2003; Breton, 1964). This clustering partially accounts for the fact that members of visible minority groups typically have fewer acquaintances outside their ethnic group than Whites (Fennema, 2004). This is particularly true for recent immigrants.

There are many different factors that affect the prevalence of residential segregation, including the city's economic base and housing types (Fong & Wilkes, 2003). Large cities with a relatively high proportion of foreign-born residents (especially recent immigrants) are also more likely to have higher levels of ethnic residential segregation (White et al., 2003). In turn, larger minority groups like the Chinese have greater resources to maintain support for "subgroup activities and institutions" (Fong & Wilkes, 2003:581) through, among other things, the accumulation of *social* and *cultural capital*. The term *social capital* is generally used to describe "social networks, the reciprocities that arise from them, and the value of these for achieving mutual goals" (Schuller, Baron, & Field, 2001:1). The concept can be used to highlight and explicate how social relations and common values influence attitudes and behaviours.

Certain ethnic groups, including the Chinese, have a history of living in relatively ethnically homogenous pockets within Canadian cities. For instance, when the Chinese first came to Canada, they were relegated to the margins of a "white man's" society (Ward, 1990). Early Chinese immigrants often lived in close proximity to one another due to rampant social discrimination (White et al., 2003). Thus, in the beginning, ethnic enclaves developed not as a means of retaining culture and identity, but as a protective response. Today residential ethnic enclaves are primarily a place of comfort and familiarity for immigrants, and they facilitate the retention of traditional aspects of culture. Within these communities, immigrants often have the support of family and can find employment and refuge in what might otherwise be an overwhelming new cultural and social context (Salaff, Fong, & Wong, 1999). The assimilation process for immigrants who join an ethnically segregated community is often much different from those who move to more ethnically diverse areas in that segregated communities more easily facilitate adherence to everyday practices (i.e., language, shopping, social interaction) that closely resemble practices from their countries of origin. Residential and community atmosphere can be very informative with respect to social patterns, structure, and relations within that society (White et al., 2003). Thus, the extent to which an ethnic enclave is *institutionally complete* may help predict whether traditional cultural ideologies and practices will be prevalent and maintained within a community.

Li (2004) argues that the effectiveness of *social capital,* defined in Chapter II as the resources gained through social relations, depends on both the breadth and depth of social ties and relations and the resources that are available to the group. Thus, *social capital's* connection to ethnic enclaves and *institutional completeness* is apparent: ethnic social ties and common values based in ethnic cultures are more easily maintained in *institutionally complete* ethnic enclaves. *Social capital* coupled with *institutional completeness* facilitates commonality between community members with respect to the beliefs they hold and the services they use (Breton, 1964; Hedley, 1980; White et al., 2003).

Li (2004:171) also stresses the fact that the creation of *social capital* "may involve a potential cost to an individual." Specifically, the ethnic attachment and the ethnic mobility entrapment theses argue that maintaining an ethnic identity and ethnic social networks actually cost individuals potential opportunities in terms of jobs and earnings. In turn, the concepts of social networks and trust are synonymous with *social capital*, and are used to help explain the connection between social relations, the resources that are gained through them, and their effect on attitudes and behaviours. The concept of *social capital* then has the ability to provide insights into how relationships, community, and social environmental factors can help improve the health and well-being of the population (Hawe & Shiell, 2000).

Research in the field of health and health care has used the notion of *social capital* to partially account for structural inequalities, such as health disparities among individuals. While good health is considered an element of *human capital, social capital* is directly related to health status (Hawe & Shiell, 2000). *Social capital* can act as a form of support. Engaging in social relations and building social networks and trust can affect health and other factors associated with general well-being (Edmondson, 2003). *Social capital* is connected to the macro-community level of health status (Hawe & Shiell, 2000). At the individual level, *social capital* and social networks work to mediate difficulties people face, whether personal, financial, or health related. In particular, social networks provide people with practical ways of coping and dealing with difficulties and structural inequality (Cattell, 2004).

Many immigrants face a multitude of barriers (e.g., language-based, cultural differences) when they attempt to access services within the health care system (Kobayashi, 2003). CAM practices provided in their first language from immigrant practitioners play an important role for some members of these communities, as barriers to access are alleviated. Because CAM practices have not been legitimated in the same way as biomedical practices, the like-mindedness of the members of these social networks also serves to legitimate the CAM practices and ideologies that are local to that particular ethnic group within that particular community. Thus, the disjuncture and inequality between CAM's position within mainstream society compared to that of biomedicine is somewhat ameliorated for immigrants who wish to engage in these practices. However, consistent with the concern Li (2004) expressed, there are potential costs as well, including the reality that immigrants who use CAM may experience stigma from people both outside and within their own ethnocultural community (Fink, 2002).

Other factors to be considered when exploring the health services and practices new immigrants use are the processes of acculturation and assimilation they undergo following their arrival in Canada. Acculturation and assimilation refer to the process wherby an individual or group of people adopts the traits of another culture (Robbins, 2005). Expectations associated with assimilation and acculturation upon arrival may have the opposite effect on immigrants who might normally use CAM. For instance, new immigrants may feel the need to be "Canadian," so they may forsake their traditional health care practices in favour of Western practices. While this may be the case in some instances, much of the literature indicates that health services are underutilized by new immigrants and that as acculturation and assimilation progresses, health service utilization increases (Salant & Lauderdale, 2003). Consistent with Satia-Abouta and her colleagues (2002) findings regarding older Chinese immigrants, Chappell and Lai found that one half of the respondents in a 1998 study continued to use TCM practices post-immigration. While it may be the case that older Chinese immigrants do not use Western care or CAM exclusively, the way in which they choose which methods they want to use is a negotiated process that takes place over time.

Finally, the presence and establishment of any formal institution's services, such as health care, increases social cohesion within the community and decreases the likelihood that people will use services outside the community, making members of an ethnic community more likely to substitute traditional ethnic practices for national ones (Breton, 1964). Two of the main measurements of *institutional completeness* are residential concentration and the provision of basic services, such as health care (Hedley, 1980). Because of the value and importance placed on customs, beliefs, and practices that are developed in a minority group's country of origin, when individuals immigrate to a new place they continue to value these same customs and beliefs, setting the stage for the creation and establishment of an *institutionally complete* community.

Due to the unavailability of many ethno-specific CAM practices in the universal health care system, members of particular visible minority communities oftentimes have to seek and pay for these services themselves, further marginalizing certain individuals and their practices and leading to the development of an underground system of unregulated and unlicensed care. The processes involved in creating an *institutionally complete* community then may directly influence members of visible minority groups and their interpersonal relationships (Breton, 1964:198).

Through this illustration of *institutionally complete* communities where levels of *social capital* are high and levels of acculturation may be low, it is apparent that ethnicity and culture guide and influence the decisions immigrants make regarding health care.

Despite the importance CAM philosophies and practices play in the lives of many immigrants, people who rely on CAM may still be nervous and ashamed to disclose to medical doctors (and sometimes family and community members due, in part, to intergenerational differences) that they use traditional/alternative forms of health care. There may be a concern that medical practitioners do not respect these health care practices, and, as a result, the patients believe they will be treated differently (Fink, 2002). Health researchers have reiterated the importance of exploring why immigrants and visible minorities use CAM so that health care professionals are better informed and able to advise and treat people accordingly (Lee, Chang, Jacobs, & Wrensch, 2002). In Western societies, the health beliefs of visible minorities are often viewed as strange, uninformed ideas resulting from a lack of knowledge about the 'facts' of modern medical science (Thorne, 1993:1931). It is important then for doctors and the medical community to be aware of their patients' health beliefs in order to provide effective diagnoses and treatment.

Chapter VII

The Effects of Immigrant Status and Ethnicity on CAM Use

Although few studies have adequately addressed the relationship between immigrant status, ethnicity, and CAM use, a rather comprehensive American study by Mackenzie and her colleagues (2003) is the first to have addressed this gap in the literature. The study involved the collection of data from a national probability sample with an over-sampling of ethnic minorities. In addition, they conducted the survey in six languages, thus expanding the number and diversity of people who were eligible for the study sample. Contrary to findings in previous studies, Mackenzie et al. (2003) found that CAM use did not vary by ethnicity. The study found that CAM use was equally likely among all ethnic groups that were included in the study. However, results did indicate that characteristics of users, including ethnicity, differed based on which form of CAM was being utilized. For example, Asians were more likely to use herbal medicines and acupuncture than any other ethnic group. Similarly, African Americans were most likely to use home remedies, and Caucasians were most likely to use chiropractic care (Mackenzie, 2003). The findings indicating that Asians were more likely than any other group to use forms of traditional Chinese medicine provide some justification for focusing on these forms of CAM in the current study.

Another study, which examined CAM use among ethnic minority older adults, found that CAM use was quite common among this group and that older immigrants are very likely to use health practices and therapies that are familiar to them. Results also confirmed that the particular form of CAM that people use varies according to ethnicity (Najm et al., 2003). Specifically,

Asians were most likely to use acupuncture and "Oriental" medicine, Hispanics dietary supplements and home remedies, and Whites chiropractic, massage, and vitamins (Najm et al., 2003). It seems that findings based on ethnicity and alternative medicine use largely depend on which CAM practices/modalities are included (or excluded) in a study. Therefore, future research in this area should consider CAM practices separately in order to obtain an accurate portrayal of CAM use among immigrants and visible minorities.

Another predictor of CAM use among visible minorities is the number of years they have lived in their new country. In Najm et al.'s (2003) study on CAM use among ethnic older adults in Orange County, California, 86.7% of those who had only been in the United States for less than a year were CAM users compared to only 45.8% of those who had lived there for more than 10 years. This indicates that time since immigration is an important factor in predicting CAM use among immigrants. Not only is it important to know why usage declines over time, but also why individuals change their patterns of CAM usage. Perhaps the most relevant finding from the Najm (2003) study in the context of the current study, however, is that ethnic minority older adults are generally more likely to rely on practices and treatments they are familiar with (often CAM) rather than those of conventional biomedicine.

In a Canadian study addressing how ethnicity affects decisions regarding health care among Chinese immigrants in Toronto, findings indicate that a multitude of problems can arise when communication barriers exist between doctors and patients (Lee, Rodin, Devins, & Weiss, 2001). As a result of these barriers, many immigrants in the study who suffered from chronic fatigue and weakness relied on self-help rather than conventional medicine. Similarly, Waxler-Morrison (2002) found that male Vietnamese medical doctors in British Columbia sometimes fail to provide information or to order testing for older Vietnamese females because of cultural beliefs these doctors hold with regard to the gendered and generational nature of health care behavior within Vietnamese culture. Another study found that patients and families typically do not question the doctor because they are perceived to have knowledge and authority in terms of health and health care (Dinh, Ganesan, & Waxler-Morrison, 1990). Additionally, many of the Chinese adults from the Lee et al. (2001) study would have preferred to consult a practitioner of traditional Chinese medicine, but due to the lack of coverage of these service(s), their use of TCM was limited.

The link between Chinese culture and the use of TCM still exists today. A limited number of studies have addressed TCM use among people of Chinese origin who have immigrated to Western countries. Ma (1999) discovered that Chinese immigrants in two major American cities were very likely to treat themselves using home remedies, and they were also fairly likely to return to their country of origin in search of care and treatment. Another study by Zhang and Verhoef (2002) concluded that when Chinese immigrants make decisions regarding disease management strategies (e.g. in this study, arthritis), they are influenced by personal and cultural factors. The study also notes that Chinese immigrants begin with self-treatment, followed by consultations with Western doctors, and then TCM practitioners before returning to Western physicians. Chinese immigrants who participated in Lee and her colleagues' 2001 study felt that TCM practitioners could better understand the true nature of their health concerns compared to a Western doctor. Unfortunately a major limitation of these studies is their lack of attention to the role that time since immigration plays in this relationship. Time since immigration is certainly important to consider since related factors, such as level of acculturation, have a significant effect on a Chinese immigrant's decision to use TCM.

Chapter VIII

Traditional Chinese Medicine

With a history dating back more than 2000 years, traditional Chinese medicine (TCM) is a long-established form of general health care, which includes diagnosis and treatment (Ou, Huang, Hampsch-Woodill, & Flanagan, 2003). The WHO officially recognizes TCM's ability to prevent, diagnose, treat, and cure many diseases and illnesses. Common TCM practices were developed through observation of their effects on specific ailments and/or parts of the body (Maciocia, 1989). Unlike the basic tenets of conventional biomedicine, TCM's theory of *yin-yang* balance has no physical meaning and is considered to be an "incomprehensible ideology" (Ou et al., 2003:1). Given this criticism, it is not surprising that the way in which TCM approaches health and health care is acknowledged as fundamentally different from that of conventional Western medicine.

In TCM, the human body is understood using a holistic view of the universe, which is rooted in Daoism. Thus, the connection between religion and TCM is implicit in the way practitioners and even patients understand health and illness. The tenets of Daoism are largely based on observing the natural world and how it operates (Kaptchuk, 2000). Moreover, TCM has two unique theories that are central to its application and implementation: the theory of *yin-yang* and the theory of five elements. In addition to these theories, TCM uses the human body meridian system as the third major component that helps substantiate its overall theoretical and philosophical framework (Maciocia, 1989).

Briefly, *yin* and *yang* represent opposites within the universe (i.e. hot/cold, fast/slow, masculine/feminine, still/moving, lower/upper etc.). *Yin* is typically characterized by, among other things, darkness, stillness, and descent, while *yang* is characterized as bright, moving, ascending, and progressing. *Yin* and *yang* are opposites and are in conflict, yet they are interdependent. A person is said to be healthy when there is a dynamic balance between *yin* and *yang* within the body. Illness and disease occur when this balance in broken. This may result from an excess or deficiency of either *yin* or *yang* (Maciocia, 1989). TCM also classifies internal organs as *yin* or *yang*. This is known as the *Zangfu* system. While each organ is recognized as having a particular function, these organs function together and have a collective capacity beyond their physiological functions outlined in Western medicine. There are five *zang* or *yin* organs, which are all solid: the spleen, the heart, the lungs, the liver, and the kidneys. There are six *fu* or *yang* organs, which are hollow: the small intestine, the large intestine, the gall bladder, the bladder, the stomach, and the *san jiao* or triple burner which is not defined in Western physiology (Maciocia, 1989).

The theory of five elements is based on a philosophical concept that is used to explain processes, functions, and other phenomena in the physical world. With regards to medicine, this theory is used to understand the relationship between the human body and the natural environment. Like *yin* and *yang*, the five elements, which include water, fire, wood, metal, and earth, are interdependent, which reflects the interconnectivity of the body and the natural environment. The interconnected promoting and restraining nature of the five elements is used to understand processes in the body. Further, each element has its own unique attributes. For example, water is characterized by moisture, cold, descending, and flowing. Fire is associated with draught, heat, flaring, ascendance, and movement, while wood is characterized by germination, extension, softness, harmony, and flexibility. Finally, metal is associated with strength, firmness, killing, and cutting, whereas earth is linked with growing, changing, nourishing, and producing. Each element is also associated with a particular season, climate, taste, colour, sound, emotion, odour, movement, sense organ, body part, and *yin* or *yang* organ (Kaptchuk, 2000).

In TCM, the human body is an energy system involving four basic vital substances, including *qi* (vital energy), *jing* (essence), blood, and body fluids. These substances are distributed throughout the body through a network of channels known as meridians. Further, there are three main causes of disharmony, which results in illness and disease. Internal causes are related to emotions, external causes are related to climatic conditions, and miscellaneous causes are related to factors, such as work, exercise, diet, and physical trauma.

TCM's diagnostic process involves four main types of examination: looking, hearing and smelling, asking, and touching (CTCMA, 2010).

There are five main treatment modalities in Chinese medicine: (1) acupuncture and moxibustion, (2) herbal therapy, (3) *tui na* (massage and manipulation), (4) therapeutic exercise (*tai chi, qi gong*), and (5) diet therapy. It is important to note that because the process of assessing an illness or condition considers the whole person, treatment is not based entirely on symptoms, thus different people may receive different treatment(s) for the same disease or condition. Likewise, different diseases and conditions may require similar treatments (Kaptchuk, 2000).

Chapter IX

Methods

Data Source and Study Sample

The data for this study are from the third wave of the CCHS, cycle 2.1 (2003), a national population health dataset. This dataset is particularly suitable for several reasons: it has a national probability sample; it is comprehensive; and, despite their under-representation, it has a relatively large number of visible minorities allowing for subgroups like the Chinese to be examined. The dataset contains 16 questions pertaining to CAM use and two main questions pertaining to ethnicity as well as characterizing information on age, gender, marital status, time since immigration, census metropolitan area, sense of belonging to local community, charter language ability, education, income, presence of chronic conditions, and health status.

The main objective of the CCHS is "to provide timely cross-sectional estimates of health determinants, health status, and health system utilization at a sub-provincial level (health region or combination of health regions)" (Statistics Canada, 2005). Data were collected in 133 health regions across Canada and in the three territories through two separate surveys: a 45 minute health region-level survey and a 60 minute provincial-level survey, both administered in 2003 through a combination of computer-assisted and personal telephone interviews. Cycle 2.1 of the CCHS consists of yes/no, Likert scaled, and multiple choice questions. The survey contains questions relating to 28 common content sections and 23 optional content sections, and was administered in English and French as well as a number of other languages. The sample is representative of household residents in all provinces and territories, with the exception of populations on Indian Reserves and Crown Lands, Canadian Forces Bases, and some remote areas. Individuals aged 12 years and older were eligible for the survey. Survey respondents were randomly selected using a probability sampling strategy (Statistics Canada, 2005).

Measures and Data Analysis

The analysis of the data was limited to the 16 questions related to CAM use, the two questions related to ethnicity, and the questions related to cultural, health, socio-demographic, and socio-economic control variables. Specifically, the CAM use variable was measured by responses to the following questions: *In the past 12 months, have you seen or talked to an alternative health care provider such as an acupuncturist, homeopath or massage therapist about your physical, emotional or mental health? If yes, who did you see or talk to - Massage therapist? Acupuncturist? Homeopath or naturopath? Feldenkraise or Alexander teacher? Relaxation therapist? Biofeedback teacher? Rolfer? Herbalist? Reflexologist? Spiritual healer? Religious healer? Other? Number of consultations tions of consualth care provider? Chiropractor?* Since there was no question that would allow us to distinguish types of users, CAM users include both those who used CAM exclusively and those who used it in combination with allopathic medicine. The questions related to ethnicity, the main independent variable, included: *People living in Canada come from many different cultural and racial backgrounds. Are [you/he/she]: White, Chinese, South Asian, Black, Filipino, Latin American, Southeast Asian, Arab, West Asian, Japanese, Korean, Aboriginal, or Other (specify); In which country [were/was] [you/he/she] born? Canada, China, France, Germany, Greece, Guyana, Hong Kong, Hungary, India, Italy, Jamaica, Netherlands/Holland, Philippines, Poland, Portugal, United Kingdom, United States, Vietnam, Sri Lanka, Other (specify).*

We analyzed the relationship between Chinese Canadian ethnicity and CAM use via Statistical Package for the Social Sciences (SPSS 13.0) software using logistic regression techniques. We also assessed the significance of immigrant status in explaining the likelihood of CAM use, after controlling for the aforementioned sociodemographic, cultural, and health variables. The dependent variable, CAM use, was dummy coded using "no" as the reference category. The main independent variable, ethnicity/racial origin, had 14 categories, and Chinese Canadian was compared to the rest of the Canadian population. Chinese ethnicity was coded as 1 and non-Chinese ethnicity as 0. The selection of control variables to be included was informed by the literature. There were four blocks of control variables: cultural; demographic; socioeconomic; and health. Aside from ethnicity, the main independent variable, the cultural variables included time since immigration, ability to converse in Canada's official languages (English and French), census metropolitan area, and sense of belonging to local community. The rationale to include these variables in the "cultural block" was based on speculation that immigrants who come from countries that adhere to alternative health ideologies, such as China, and who relocate to urban areas that have at least partially *institutionally complete* communities may have a higher probability of using CAM compared to other Canadians.

The demographic variables tested included age, gender, and marital status, while the socioeconomic variables included education and income. According to previous studies (see Eisenberg et al., 1998; Eisenberg et al, 1993; Millar, 1997; McFarland et al., 2002), age, gender, marital status, education, and income all have significant effects on CAM use within the general population; therefore, we speculated that these factors may be predictors for Chinese Canadians as well. Given their demographic profile, Chinese Canadians in this sample were also likely to be immigrants (foreign-born). The census metropolitan area variable provided a geographic marker with which to measure the level of *institutional completeness* in certain communities within cities. The sense of belonging to community variable was coded as "weak" (somewhat weak or very weak) and "strong" (somewhat strong or very strong) based on the question: *How would you describe your sense of belonging to your local community? Would you say it is (very strong, somewhat strong, somewhat weak, or very weak?* Finally, the health variables included self-reported health status and the presence of a chronic condition/illness. Canadians are more likely to use CAM when they are suffering from a chronic illness. Presumably, if the same correlation holds for Chinese Canadians, this may provide further insight into why Chinese Canadians use CAM. The self-reported health status variable was coded as "positive" (excellent, very good, or good) or "negative" (fair or poor) based on the question: *In general, would you say your health is (excellent, very good, good, fair, or poor)?* The chronic condition variable, coded Yes/No, was derived from 31 other variables. [See the CCHS documentation on data and derived variables for further information] (Statistics Canada, 2005).

Missing cases were dealt with in a number of ways. In some instances where missing cases (including those who responded with "Not Stated") comprised a substantial proportion of cases within the variable, they were made into a new category within the variable. Specifically, the missing cases for education and income were included as an additional category called "Missing." The "Not Applicable" category from the time since immigration variable represents people who have not immigrated, so these cases were used to create a reference category: "Canadian-Born." Finally, if there were very few missing cases within the variable, which was the case for CAM use, ethnicity, language ability, census metropolitan area, sense of belonging to community, marital status, age, self-reported health status, and presence of a chronic condition, these cases were left out of the analysis. In total, 8,827 of a possible 135,573 cases were excluded from the analysis for an overall sample size of 126,746 for all Canadians. The sample size for the Chinese subs-sample was 2,146, with 179 cases of a possible 2,325 excluded. The percentage of missing cases was 6.5% and 7.7% respectively, slightly above the informal "rule" of 5.0%. The analyses were run with and without the missing cases. Since there was essentially no difference between the results, the higher proportion of missing cases was excluded to allow for a more coherent interpretation of the results.

Chapter X

Results

Sample Characteristics

Table 1 provides descriptive statistics for each study variable within the two samples: (1) all Canadians and (2) Chinese Canadians. In the sample that includes all Canadians, 12.4% of respondents report using CAM within the past year. The sample of all Canadians is 3.8% Chinese and 96.2% non-Chinese. Most respondents are Canadian-born (79.4%), while the rest are either recent (5.5%) or long-term (15.1%) immigrants. Only 2.0% of the overall sample cannot speak either English or French. The majority of respondents live in a census metropolitan area (CMA). Specifically, 16.2% of the sample lives in Toronto, 6.9% in Vancouver, and 42.2% in another CMA, while 34.7% of respondents do not live in a CMA. Almost two-thirds (63.9%) of respondents reported having a strong sense of belonging to their local community compared to only 36.1% who reported a weak sense of belonging. The gender distribution is 49.3% male and 50.7% female. Over one half of respondents are either married or living common law (58.3%), while 30.0% are single, 6.7% are separated or divorced, and 5.0% are widowed. The mean age of the sample is 42.6 years. Almost one half of the sample (46.4%) have completed a post-secondary degree, while 7.6% have completed some post-secondary education, 17.8% have finished high school, and 26.1% have less than a high school education. Income ranges from low to high, with more than three quarters of respondents falling into the middle, upper-middle, and high income categories. An overwhelming majority (88.7%) self-report positive health status (excellent, very good, or good) contrasted with 11.3% who report

negative health status (fair or poor). Despite this, 68.6% of respondents suffer
from at least one chronic illness.

**Table 1. Descriptive Information for CAM Use, Cultural, Socio-
demographic, Socio-economic, and Health Variables by All Canadians
and Chinese Canadians Only**

Variable	All Canadians Sample N = 135,573 % (N)	Chinese Only Sample N = 2,325 % (N)
CAM use		
Yes	12.4% (16,774)	14.9% (345)
No	87.6% (118,720)	85.1% (1,978)
Ethnicity		
Chinese	3.8% (4,930)	100.0% (2,325)
Non-Chinese	96.2% (126,307)	0.0% (0)
Time Since Immigration		
0-9 Years	5.5% (7,189)	31.6% (726)
10+ Years	15.1% (19,860)	48.4% (1,112)
Canadian-Born	79.4% (104,167)	20.0% (461)
Language		
English/French	98.0% (128,837)	80.9% (1,882)
No English/French	2.0% (2663)	19.1% (443)
Census Metropolitan Area		
Other	42.2% (57,257)	20.6% (479)
Toronto	16.2% (21,922)	42.2% (982)
Vancouver	6.9% (9,403)	34.5% (802)
None	34.7% (46,990)	2.7% (63)
Sense of Belonging to Community		
Weak	36.1% (47,224)	46.2% (1,018)
Strong	63.9% (83,485)	53.8% (1,183)
Gender		
Male	49.3% (66,773)	47.9% (1,115)
Female	50.7% (68,800)	52.1% (1,210)
Marital Status		
Married/Common Law	58.3%(78,972)	57.6% (1,337)
Widowed	5.0% (6,779)	3.4% (78)
Separated/Divorced	6.7% (9,013)	2.8% (66)
Single	30.0% (40,593)	36.2% (840)
Education		
Post-Secondary	46.4% (62,960)	46.4% (1,078)
Some Post-Secondary	7.6% (10,272)	8.8% (204)
High School	17.8% (24,123)	19.9% (463)
< High School	26.1% (35,376)	21.8% (506)

Variable	All Canadians Sample N = 135,573 % (N)	Chinese Only Sample N = 2,325 % (N)
Missing	2.1% (2,842)	3.2% (75)
Income		
Low	2.4% (3,213)	5.3% (124)
Lower-middle	5.2% (7,007)	7.3% (170)
Middle	16.5% (22,308)	19.5% (452)
Upper-middle	28.6% (38,782)	23.7% (552)
High	30.5% (41,417)	22.9% (533)
Missing	16.9% (22,845)	21.2% (493)
Age	42.57 (12-104)	39.18 (12-96)
Self-reported Health Status		
Positive	88.7% (120,111)	86.9% (2,021)
Negative	11.3% (15,369)	13.1% (304)
Chronic Condition		
Yes	68.6% (92,757)	53.5% (1,234)
No	31.4% (42,417)	46.5% (1,071)

In contrast, the distributions for each variable in the Chinese Canadian sample are quite different from those in the all-Canadian sample. For example, 14.9% of Chinese Canadians used some form of CAM within the past year. This is higher than the reported use among all Canadians. The three most common CAM modalities among Chinese Canadians are acupuncture, massage therapy, and herbalists. Unlike the sample that includes all Canadians, most of the people in the Chinese Canadian sample are immigrants: 31.6% are recent immigrants, 48.4% are long term immigrants, and only 20.0% are Canadian-born. A large majority (over 97.0%) of Chinese Canadians sampled live in a CMA, with most living in Toronto (42.2%) and Vancouver (34.5%). Chinese Canadians' sense of belonging to their local community is split almost evenly with 53.8% reporting a strong sense of belonging compared to 46.2% who report a weak sense of belonging. The Chinese sample has more women (52.1%) than men (47.9%). Similar to the overall Canadian sample, most Chinese Canadians are either married/living common law (57.6%) or single (36.2%). The average age within the Chinese Canadian sample is 39.2 years. The education distribution is also very similar to that of the overall Canadian sample: most have a post-secondary education (46.4%), 21.8% have less than a high school diploma, 19.9% are high school graduates, and 8.8% have completed some post-secondary education. Similarly, most Chinese Canadians report middle, upper-middle, or high incomes. However, the proportion of Chinese Canadians in the low (5.3%) and lower-middle (7.3%) income range is considerably higher than the overall Canadian sample.

The distributions for the health variables are also similar. A large majority of Chinese Canadians self-report positive health status (86.9%), whereas 13.1% report negative health status. However, 53.5% of Chinese Canadians within the sample report having at least one chronic illness, much lower than the overall Canadian sample (68.6%).

Logistic Regression Results: CAM Use among All Canadians

Table 2 presents the logistic regression results from the analysis of CAM use within the Canadian population. The logistic regression analyses reveal that Chinese Canadians are more likely to use CAM than non-Chinese Canadians, even after controlling for cultural, socio-demographic, socio-economic, and health status differences. Indeed, Chinese Canadians are more than 1.5 times more likely (p<0.001) to report having consulted an alternative health care provider than non-Chinese Canadians.

The cultural variables also influence respondents' likelihood of using CAM. Within the overall Canadian population, immigrants are less likely to use CAM than the Canadian-born. Interestingly, longer term immigrants' likelihood of using CAM (OR=0.77; p<0.001) more closely resembles that of the Canadian-born compared to recent immigrants (OR=0.51; p<0.001). Aside from respondents who reside in Vancouver, living in a census metropolitan area (CMA) does not have a significant effect on predicting CAM use. Vancouverites are 1.2 times more likely (p<0.001) than people who do not reside in a CMA to report having used CAM; however, language and sense of belonging to community do not have significant effects on predicting use.

Socio-demographic and socio-economic factors are also key in predicting CAM use. Specifically, with regard to gender, men (OR=0.47; p<0.001) are far less likely to use CAM than women. In terms of SES, the likelihood of using CAM also increases as respondents' level of education increases; that is, post-secondary graduates (OR=2.14; p<0.001), people with some post secondary education (OR=1.69; p<0.001), and high school graduates (OR=1.39; p<0.001) are all considerably more likely to report having used CAM than respondents who have less than a high school diploma. Correspondingly, higher income also results in a greater likelihood of using

CAM. Lower income (OR=0.48; p<0.001), lower middle income (OR=0.54; p<0.001), middle income (OR=0.63; p<0.001), and upper middle income (OR=0.80; p<0.001) respondents all have lower odds of using CAM than respondents from the highest income category. The age squared coefficient indicates that the effect of age is non-linear, with CAM use peaking in midlife, between 40 and 55 years of age. Marital status is not a significant predictor of use.

Table 2. Odds Ratios with 95% Confidence Intervals (C.I.) for CAM Use by Ethnicity, Cultural, Socio-demographic, Socio-economic, and Health Status Controls (Logistic Regression)

	Model 1	Model 2	Model 3	Model 4
Ethnicity				
Chinese	1.24*	1.44*	1.50*	1.58*
(95% C.I.)	(1.14, 1.34)	(1.31, 1.58)	(1.37, 1.65)	(1.43, 1.74)
Non-Chinese	1.00	1.00	1.00	1.00
Time Since Immigration				
0-9 years		0.47*	0.46*	0.51*
(95% C.I.)		(0.42, 0.51)	(0.42, 0.51)	(0.46, 0.56)
10+ years		0.76*	0.75*	0.77*
(95% C.I.)		(0.72, 0.80)	(0.71, 0.80)	(0.73, 0.81)
Canadian-Born		1.00	1.00	1.00
Language				
No English/ French		0.93	1.34*	1.36*
(95% C.I.)		(0.81, 1.08)	(1.16, 1.56)	(1.17, 1.58)
English and/or French		1.00	1.00	1.00
Census Metropolitan Area				
Toronto		1.17*	1.00	0.98
(95% C.I.)		(1.11, 1.24)	(0.94, 1.05)	(0.93, 1.04)
Vancouver		1.39*	1.21*	1.20*
(95% C.I.)		(1.29, 1.49)	(1.13, 1.30)	(1.12, 1.29)
Other		1.18*	1.05*	1.05*
(95% C.I.)		(1.14, 1.23)	(1.01, 1.09)	(1.01, 1.09)
None		1.00	1.00	1.00
Sense of Belonging to Community				
Weak		1.07*	1.04*	1.02
(95% C.I.)	(1.04, 1.11)	(1.00, 1.08)	(0.99, 1.06)	
Strong		1.00	1.00	1.00

Table 2. (Continued).

	Model 1	Model 2	Model 3	Model 4
Gender				
Male			0.45*	0.47*
(95% C.I.)			(0.44, 0.47)	(0.45, 0.49)
Female			1.00	1.00
Marital Status				
Married/Common Law			0.98	0.99
(95% C.I.)			(0.93, 1.04)	(0.94, 1.04)
Widowed			0.92	0.93
(95% C.I.)			(0.80, 1.04)	(0.82, 1.05)
Separated/Divorced			1.13*	1.12*
(95% C.I.)			(1.04, 1.22)	(1.04, 1.22)
Single			1.00	1.00
Education				
Post Secondary Graduate			2.10*	2.14*
(95% C.I.)			(1.98, 2.22)	(2.02, 2.26)
Some Post Secondary			1.68*	1.69*
(95% C.I.)			(1.55, 1.82)	(1.56,1.83)
High School Graduate			1.36*	1.39*
(95% C.I.)			(1.28, 1.46)	(1.30, 1.48)
Missing			1.66*	1.70*
(95% C.I.)			(1.44, 1.91)	(1.47, 1.96)
< High School			1.00	1.00
Income				
Lower			0.50*	0.48*
(95% C.I.)			(0.44, 0.58)	(0.41, 0.55)
Lower Middle			0.57*	0.54*
(95% C.I.)			(0.52, 0.63)	(0.49, 0.60)
Middle			0.64*	0.63*
(95% C.I.)			(0.61, 0.68)	(0.59, 0.66)
Upper Middle			0.81*	0.80*
(95% C.I.)			(0.78, 0.84)	(0.77, 0.84)
Missing			0.67*	0.67*
(95% C.I.)			(0.63, 0.72)	(0.63, 0.71)
Highest			1.00	1.00
Age			1.08*	1.08*
(95% C.I.)			(1.07, 1.09)	(1.07, 1.09)

	Model 1	Model 2	Model 3	Model 4
Age Squared			1.00*	1.00*
Self Reported Health Status				
Positive				0.86*
(95% C.I.)				(0.81, 0.91)
Negative				1.00
Chronic Condition				
Yes				1.70*
(95% C.I.)				(1.63, 1.78)
No				1.00
Model Chi Square	<0.001	<0.001	<0.001	<0.001
Cox & Snell R-Square	<0.001	0.004	0.049	0.094
Nagelkerke R-Square	<0.001	0.007	0.092	0.102
N =	131,780	127,297	127,094	126,746

Respondents who self-reported positive health status (OR=0.86; p<0.001) are less likely to use CAM than those who reported negative health status. In addition, people who suffer from at least one chronic condition (OR=1.70; p<0.001) are considerably more likely to report having used CAM than people who do not have any chronic conditions.

Logistic Regression Results: CAM Use among Chinese Canadians

Table 3 presents logistic regression results from the analysis of CAM use among Chinese Canadians. While some of the cultural variables, including time since immigration and language, are not statistically significant, sense of belonging to local community and living in one of two major CMAs are key predictors of use. Chinese Canadians who have a weak sense of belonging to community (OR=0.75; p=0.036) are less likely to use CAM than Chinese respondents who feel strongly connected. Further, Chinese Canadians who reside in Toronto (OR=2.74; p=0.055) or Vancouver (OR=3.40; p=0.021) are considerably more likely to use CAM than Chinese Canadians who do not live in a CMA.

Table 3. Odds Ratios and 95% Confidence Intervals (C.I.) for CAM Use of Chinese Canadians by Cultural, Socio-demographic, Socio-economic, and Health Status Controls (Logistic Regression)

	Model 1	Model 2	Model 3
Time Since Immigration			
0-9 years	1.37	0.86	0.93
(95% C.I.)	(0.92, 2.04)	(0.55, 1.35)	(0.59, 1.47)
10+ years	1.98*	1.06	1.06
(95% C.I.)	(1.38, 2.85)	(0.70, 1.61)	(0.70, 1.62)
Canadian-Born	1.00	1.00	0.00
Language			
No English/French	1.07	1.01	0.99
(95% C.I.)	(0.79, 1.46)	(0.70, 1.45)	(0.68, 1.44)
English and/or French	1.00	1.00	1.00
Census Metropolitan Area			
Toronto	2.10	2.66	2.74
(95% C.I.)	(0.77, 5.70)	(0.96, 7.39)	(0.98, 7.67)
Vancouver	2.74*	3.25*	3.36*
(95% C.I.)	(1.01, 7.46)	(1.17, 9.06)	(1.20, 9.42)
Other	1.55	1.81	1.83
(95% C.I.)	(0.56, 4.35)	(0.63, 5.16)	(0.64, 5.26)
None	1.00	1.00	1.00
Sense of Belonging to Community			
Weak	0.74*	0.77	0.75*
(95% C.I.)	(0.58, 0.95)	(0.60, 1.00)	(0.58, 0.98)
Strong	1.00	1.00	1.00
Gender			
Male		0.46*	0.48*
(95% C.I.)		(0.36, 0.60)	(0.37, 0.63)
Female		1.00	1.00
Marital Status			
Married/Common Law		1.20	1.18
(95% C.I.)		(0.77, 1.88)	(0.75, 1.86)
Widowed		2.45	2.34
(95% C.I.)		(0.95, 6.31)	(0.90, 6.05)
Separated/Divorced		1.47	1.42
(95% C.I.)		(0.72, 3.02)	(0.68, 2.95)
Single		1.00	1.00

	Model 1	Model 2	Model 3
Education			
Post Secondary Graduate		1.39	1.49
(95% C.I.)		(0.91, 2.12)	(0.97, 2.29)
Some Post Secondary		0.91	0.91
(95% C.I.)		(0.47, 1.77)	(0.46, 1.78)
High School Graduate		1.85*	2.00*
(95% C.I.)		(1.19, 2.87)	(1.28, 3.11)
Missing		2.43*	2.82*
(95% C.I.)		(1.16, 5.11)	(1.33, 5.96)
< High School		1.00	1.00
Income			
Lower		0.65	0.66
(95% C.I.)		(0.31, 1.38)	(0.31, 1.40)
Lower Middle		1.44	1.45
(95% C.I.)		(0.85, 2.43)	(0.85, 2.47)
Middle		0.95	0.95
(95% C.I.)		(0.63, 1.42)	(0.63, 1.43)
Upper Middle		1.45*	1.50*
(95% C.I.)		(1.01, 2.09)	(1.04, 2.15)
Missing		0.97	0.98
(95% C.I.)		(0.64, 1.49)	(0.64, 1.51)
Highest		1.00	1.00
Age		1.13*	1.13*
(95% C.I.)		(1.07, 1.20)	(1.06, 1.20)
Age Squared		1.00*	1.00*
Self Reported Health Status			
Positive			0.67*
(95% C.I.)			(0.46, 0.97)
Negative			1.00
Chronic Condition			
Yes			1.64*
(95% C.I.)			(1.24, 2.17)
No			1.00
Model Chi-Square	<0.001	<0.001	<0.001
Cox & Snell R-Square	0.018	0.071	0.080
Nagelkerke R-Square	0.033	0.126	0.142
N=	2,168	2,164	2,146

Similar to the cultural variables, many of the socio-demographic and socio-economic variables are not significant predictors of CAM use among the Chinese Canadian population. In particular, marital status, education (with the exception of high school graduates), and income are not statistically significant. In contrast, gender is an important predictor of CAM use. Chinese men (OR=0.48; p<0.001) are much less likely to use CAM than women, which is consistent with the findings from the larger sample with all Canadians. Again, the effect of age is non-linear with Chinese Canadians use of CAM peaking between the ages of 50 and 65 years – in the latter years of mid-life.

Akin to the results for all Canadians, having positive self-reported health status (OR=0.67; p=0.033) lowers the odds of using, while the presence of a chronic condition increases a Chinese respondent's likelihood of using CAM more than 1.6 times (p=0.001). In sum, the key predictors of CAM use among the Chinese Canadian population are a strong sense of belonging to local community, living in a census metropolitan area (i.e., Toronto or Vancouver), being female, being between 50 and 65 years of age, having negative health status, and suffering from at least one chronic condition.

Exploring Intersectionality: Interaction Results

There are two statistically significant three-way interactions from the sample of all Canadians that are particularly relevant to this study. Both models are significant at the p<0.001 level. Consistent with earlier findings from the full model in the all-Canadian sample, the three-way interaction between ethnicity, time since immigration, and gender confirmed that Chinese Canadians have considerably higher odds of using CAM than non-Chinese Canadians; in addition, it also establishes that women are much more likely to use CAM than men in both the Chinese Canadian and non-Chinese Canadian populations. However, the interaction also reveals that this gender difference is much stronger among Chinese Canadians, especially for the foreign born. Immigrant Chinese women have significantly higher odds of using CAM than any other group, including non-Chinese immigrants and both Chinese and non-Chinese Canadian-born respondents.[3] Specifically, for recent Chinese

---

[3] The odds ratios from the interaction between ethnicity, time since immigration, and gender should be interpreted using non-Chinese, Canadian-born women as the reference group. Their odds ratio is 1.00.

immigrants, the difference between males (0.45) and females (1.21) is 0.76. Within the non-Chinese population of recent immigrants, this difference is marginal, with men (0.24) remaining less likely to report having used CAM than women (0.39). This gender difference is even more apparent among long-term Chinese immigrants, where women have odds of 1.48 compared to 0.59 for men. Finally, one other interesting difference is that CAM use differs very little between Canadian-born male and female Chinese. Conversely, non-Chinese Canadian-born men and women differ substantially, with women (1.00) being much more likely than men (0.46) to have reported using CAM.

Ethnicity*Time Since Immigration*Gender

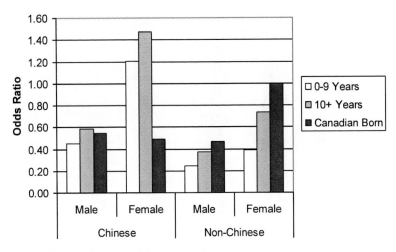

Figure 1. Three-Way Interaction between Ethnicity, Time Since Immigration, and Gender Predicting Odds of CAM use.

The results from the interaction between ethnicity, census metropolitan area, and sense of belonging to local community are interesting in the context of the literature on ethnicity and *social capital*.[4] Having a strong sense of belonging to the local community has more of an effect on Chinese Canadians living in either Toronto or Vancouver compared to any other group. In fact, Chinese Canadians who feel strongly connected to their communities and who live in Vancouver have the highest odds of using CAM (2.78), while those

---

[4] Odds ratios for this interaction, between ethnicity, time since immigration, and sense of belonging to the local community, should be interpreted in reference to non-Chinese Canadians who have a strong sense of belonging to their local community and who do not live in a census metropolitan area. They have an odds ratio of 1.00.

with the same characteristics who live in Toronto also have very high odds (2.23). Chinese Canadians who feel weakly connected to their communities have much lower odds of using CAM, especially if they reside outside of either Toronto or Vancouver. Sense of belonging to the local community does not seem to have much of an effect on the likelihood of CAM use among non-Chinese Canadians. Indeed, in some cases, non-Chinese Canadians who feel weakly connected to their local community have slightly higher odds of using CAM than their strongly connected counterparts.

Ethnicity*Sense of Belonging to Community*Census Metropolitan Area

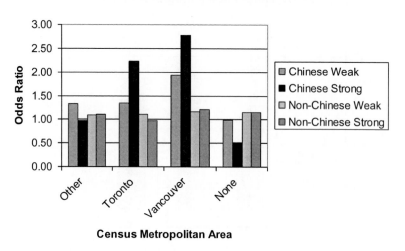

Figure 2. Three-Way Interaction between Ethnicity, Sense of Belonging to Community, and Census Metropolitan Area Predicting Odds of CAM use.

Discussion

Although Chinese Canadians are more likely to use alternative medicine than non-Chinese Canadians, ethnicity alone may not be able to entirely account for this difference. Cultural factors relating to ethnicity however, begin to account for this discrepancy. The fact that two of the three most commonly sought CAM modalities (acupuncture and herbalist) used by Chinese Canadians are rooted in traditional Chinese medicine speaks to the cultural aspects of use. Interestingly, length of time since immigration and official language ability are not statistically significant predictors of CAM use for Chinese Canadians. This is somewhat surprising given that two other culturally related variables -- i.e., census metropolitan area and sense of belonging to local community -- are, in fact, key predictors of use among Chinese Canadians. It is important to note, however, that time since immigration is significant for Chinese Canadians until the socio-demographic and socio-economic control variables are added to the model. This lack of statistical significance after controls are introduced then may be the result of more salient predictors, such as census metropolitan area and sense of belonging to local community, and a relatively small sample size of Chinese Canadians, especially Canadian-born Chinese. Further, the inability to converse in either English or French may have resulted in the exclusion of many potential ethnic Chinese participants from the CCHS given that a very small number of Statistics Canada interviewers for this iteration of the survey were able to converse in a Chinese dialect(s). Insights into such exclusion are important given that language (in)ability is paramount in being able to access health care for ethnic minority adults within the Canadian system regardless of place of residence (Kobayashi, 2003).

Consistent with the literature regarding the relationship between *institutional completeness* and *social capital*, Chinese Canadians who live in Toronto or Vancouver and who feel strongly connected to their local communities have higher odds of using CAM. This may indicate that, compared to other parts of Canada, Toronto and Vancouver have more *institutionally complete* Chinese Canadian communities within their greater metropolitan areas. Specifically, this could mean that CAM services are more readily available and that use of such services are more "socially and culturally acceptable," at least within the relatively large number of Chinese Canadian communities in these two cities. This possible explanation is further confirmed by the fact that these two variables, living in a CMA and feeling connected to local community, are not nearly as salient in predicting CAM use among non-Chinese Canadians. Finally, since very little research on CAM has focused on utilization patterns among ethno-cultural minorities, it is extremely difficult to verify these findings with previous research. Qualitative data derived from in-depth face-to-face interviews with Chinese Canadians may also help us to make further sense of these findings.

With respect to socio-demographic and socio-economic variables functioning as predictors of CAM use, the current study's findings corroborate major findings from previous studies (Eisenberg et al, 1998; Eisenberg et al, 1993; Millar, 1997). Specifically, the study found that users tend to be women who have a relatively high education and income, and that, on average,

Canadian users (40-55 years) tend to be slightly younger than Chinese Canadian users (50-65 years).

Regardless of ethnicity, women are more likely to use CAM than men. This is consistent with findings from previous research, which concludes that women tend to utilize health care services more than men (Segall & Chappell, 2000). While both Chinese and non-Chinese women are more likely to use CAM than men, gender is the only variable that has almost the same effect in both the overall Canadian sample and the Chinese Canadian sample. Unlike findings from previous studies and the overall Canadian sample in this study, income and education are not key predictors of CAM use for Chinese Canadians. While this may be a function of the relatively small sample size, it is still a noteworthy finding. Nonetheless, because adherence to traditional forms of Chinese medicine is generally accepted within the Chinese Canadian community and given the cultural importance of maintaining traditional values and beliefs, perhaps the relative unimportance of education and income – two key predictors for typical Western CAM users – can be explained by the fact that other predictors related to culture are more salient for the Chinese. For non-Chinese Canadians, the decision to consult an alternative medical practitioner may largely depend on their financial ability to access these services, while such a factor may not be as important for Chinese Canadians. This makes sense given that previous research indicates that health beliefs and their etiology have a major impact on the type of care people seek (Hellman, 1991).

As a predictor, the role of health status appears to be similar for respondents from both samples given that negative self-reported health status and the presence of a chronic condition increase the likelihood of using CAM. This speaks to the overall importance of health status (both subjective and objective) in predicting CAM use regardless of other factors.

Finally, the significant three-way interactions indicate that certain identity markers must be combined for their full predictive value to be revealed. The interactions allow for deeper insights into how specific variables may operate/intersect in predicting CAM use in addition to providing important insights into Chinese Canadians' reasons for such use.

The interaction between ethnicity, time since immigration, and gender indicates that Chinese immigrant women are more likely to use CAM than all males, non-Chinese females, and all those who are Canadian-born. Interestingly, time since immigration was not statistically significant within the Chinese sample, which can be partially attributed to the interaction between the three variables since gender and ethnicity appear to be extremely important in predicting CAM use. Chinese immigrant women may be more likely to hold traditional understandings of health and illness that are more consistent with health care practitioners in countries like China, Hong Kong, or Taiwan, where "exposure" to such "alternative" (traditional) health beliefs and practices is high. If so, this interaction demonstrates that these women may be more inclined to use a combination of CAM and Western medicine.

The second interaction between ethnicity, census metropolitan area, and sense of belonging to community is also very interesting and complex. Chinese Canadians who live in either Toronto or Vancouver and who feel strongly connected to their local community are much more likely to use alternative medicine than both non-Chinese respondents and Chinese respondents who feel weakly connected to their communities or who do not reside in either Toronto or Vancouver. This interaction indicates that having a strong sense of belonging to community only results in higher odds of CAM use for Chinese respondents who live in either Toronto or Vancouver. Perhaps Chinese respondents living in more *institutionally complete* communities in Toronto and Vancouver have higher levels of *social capital* which translates into feeling more connected to their communities via an increased sense of support from friends and family members to use alternative services. Such speculation, however, requires further examination using other exploratory methods. Indeed, qualitative data can be used to expound upon these interpretations to paint a more comprehensive picture of utilization patterns, experiences, and reasons for use among Canada's Chinese population.

Regardless of the support qualitative data may provide to the study's findings, the current results are important on their own in the context of policy and program development vis-à-vis alternative health services for visible minority immigrant Canadians. Specifically, the findings speak to the importance of improving access to and the delivery of culturally sensitive care to Chinese Canadian immigrants. One way this can be done, for example, is through the education of Western physicians about Chinese medicine and other forms of CAM so as to increase appreciation, understanding, and acceptance of other forms of health care in policy and practise.

Further, in confirming that Chinese Canadians are, in fact, more likely to use CAM than non-Chinese Canadians, we realize that the improvement of culturally sensitive care may also be done through the promotion of "mainstreaming;" that is, the creation of health policy and programs that acknowledge and include understandings of ethnicity and culture to help alleviate inequality, especially at the individual level, through the validation of traditional health beliefs, while continuing to promote integration into

Canadian society. An adoption of "mainstreaming" programs does not necessarily mean that Chinese medicine services should be covered under the universal system; rather, through new policy and program directives, there needs to be open acknowledgment of differences related to deeply-rooted cultural aspects of identity and the often unacknowledged barriers to access to Western care. Such acknowledgement may assist in validating the traditional views of immigrant TCM users and promote improved access to Western health care. Efforts to recognize the source of barriers to accessing care (i.e., traditional understandings of health) rather than the indicators of these barriers, such as language, are certainly in order.

Limitations

In conclusion, a few limitations of this study should be highlighted. First, the way the CCHS defines CAM is limited in that it does not clearly acknowledge the diversity vis-à-vis power, mandate, and regulation (and their inter-relationships) between various forms of CAM. At a minimum, a more complete definition of CAM should separate modalities based on standards such as regulation and licensing. Without this, the CCHS definition fails to acknowledge that certain CAM modalities, like chiropractic care, massage therapy, and midwifery, may be perceived (and therefore treated) differently by allopathic doctors and Canadian health care users compared to TCM, for example. A more comprehensive definition that addresses this issue would perhaps help to differentiate between more and less "legitimate" forms of CAM, which, in turn, would provide further insights into who (i.e., the demographic profiles of users) uses different forms of CAM.

Second, given that visible minorities and immigrants are underrepresented in the CCHS, the findings may have been limited due to the small sample size of Canadian-born versus foreign-born Chinese. Further, small sample sizes made comparison between specific Chinese groups (i.e. Canadian-born, Mainland Chinese, Taiwanese, etc.) difficult. Third, the measures for *social capital* (the sense of belonging to local community variable) and *institutional completeness* (the census metropolitan area variable) were limited by how these concepts were operationalized according to CCHS survey questions. The sense of belonging variable is subject to the respondent's interpretation with respect to whether he or she characterizes "local community" as ethnic, physical neighbourhood, or a variation of these. Although this variable has been used as a measure for *social capital* in previous Canadian studies, it may be limited in its ability to specify how connected people feel to their ethnocultural community. Further, while living in one of many *institutionally complete* communities in Toronto or Vancouver (e.g., Markham, Richmond) may have an impact on the utilization of CAM, it is also important to acknowledge that these communities vary demographically and politically, so presumably the ways in which they impact TCM use may vary as well. Therefore, the census metropolitan variable is limited because it is unable to account for differences between these communities, differences that may affect utilization patterns. It is recommended that the census metropolitan variable be broken down further into postal code districts, which would provide a more accurate measure of *institutionally complete* communities within larger urban centres like Toronto and Vancouver.

Future Research

Based on a extensive review of the literature and the findings from this central study, it is recommended that future research in this area focus on specific types of CAM practices since broad definitions of CAM are often inconsistent across studies. Consistency across definitions would facilitate the ability to make cross-comparisons with other studies. Further, exploratory qualitative research with a diverse sample of Chinese Canadians would offer further insights into the reasons *why* there is a connection between Chinese Canadian ethnicity and CAM use. In addition, replicating this study by focusing on different Chinese Canadian groups (i.e., Canadian-born and immigrants from Mainland China, Taiwan, Hong Kong, etc.) would provide further insights into differences in utilization patterns between these groups and would serve to acknowledge the diversity that exists within the Chinese Canadian population by country of origin.

References

Alund, A. 2003. "Ethnicity, social subordination, and cultural resistance." *Comparative Social Research*. Vol. 22. Pp. 245-261.

Astin, J. 1998. "Why patients use alternative medicine: results of a national study." *Journal of the American Medical Association*. Vol 279. No. 19. pp. 1548-1553.

Bair, Y., Gale, E., Greendale, G., Sternfeld, B., Adler, S., Azari, R., & M. Harkey, 2002. "Ethnic Differences in Use of Complementary and Alternative Medicine at Midlife: Longitudinal Results from SWAN participants." *American Journal of Public Health*. Vol. 92. No. 11. pp. 1832-1841.

Barnes, PM ., Bloom, B., and RL Nahin. 2008. "Complementary and alternative medicine use among adults and children: United States, 2007" *National Health Statistics Report*. No. 12. pp. 1-23.

Bates, DG. 2000. "Why not call modern medicine 'alternative?'" *Perspectives in Biology and Medicine*. Vol. 34. No. 4. pp. 502-518.

Bodeker, G. & F. Kronenberg. 2002. "A public health agenda for traditional, complementary, and alternative medicine." *American Journal of Public Health*. Vol. 92. No. 10. pp. 1582-1591.

Boon, HS., Verhoef, MJ., Vanderheyden, LC., & KP Westlake. 2006. "Complementary and alternative medicine: a rising healthcare issue. *Healthcare Policy*. Vol 1. No. 3. pp. 19-30.

Bourdieu, P. 1997. "The Forms of Capital." Pp.46-58 in A. Halsey et al. (eds.). *Education: Culture, Economy, and Society*. New York: Oxford University Press.

Breton, R. 1964. "Institutional completeness of ethnic communities and personal relations to immigrants." *American Journal of Sociology*. Vol 70. pp.193-205.

Canadian College of Naturopathic Medicine. 2010. "Principles of Naturapathic Medicine." Available from: http://www.ccnm.edu/about_ccnm/principles_naturopathic_medicine

Cattel, V. 2004. "Social Networks as Mediators between the Harsh Circumstances of Lives, and Their Lived Experience of Health and Well-Being." pp. 142-161 in Phillipson et al. (eds.). *Social Networks and Social Exclusion: Sociological and Policy Perspectives*. Aldershot: Ashgate.

College of Traditional Chinese Medicine Practitioners and Acupuncturists of British Columbia. 2010. Available from: http://www.ctcma.bc.ca

Conrad, P. 1992. "Medicalization and Social Control." *Annual Review of Sociology*. Vol. 18. pp. 209-232.

Dinh, D., Ganesan, S. & N. Waxler-Morrison, 1990. "The Vietnamese." Pp. 181-213 in N. Waxler-Morrison et al. (eds.). *Cross-Cultural Caring: A Handbook for Professionals in Western Canada*. Vancouver: University of British Columbia Press.

Department of Justice Canada. 2010. Canadian Multiculturalism Act 1985." Available from: http://laws.justice.gc.ca/eng/C-18.7/page-1.html

Edmondson, R. 2003. "Social Capital: A Strategy for Enhancing Health?" *Social Science & Medicine*. Vol. 57. pp. 1723-1733.

Eisenberg, D., Davis, R., Ettner, S., Appel, S., Wilkey, S., Van Rompay, M., and R. Kessler. 1998. "Trends in alternative medicine use in the United States, 1990-1997: results of a follow-up national survey." *Journal of the American Medical Association*. Vol. 280. No.18. pp. 1569-1575.

Eisenberg, D., Kessler, R., Foster, C., Norlock, F., Calkins, D. & T. Delbanco. 1993. "Unconventional Medicine in the United States – Prevalence, Costs, and Patterns of Use." *New England Journal of Medicine*, Vol. 328. No. 4. pp. 246-252.

Evans, RG. 1994. "Introduction." Pp. 3-26 in RG. Evans, ML. Barer, & TR. Marmor (eds.). *Why are some people healthy and others not? The determinants of health of populations*. New York: Aldine de Gruyter.

Evans RG. & GL. 1994. "Producing health, consuming health care." pp. 27-64 in RG. Evans, ML. Barer, & TR. Marmor (eds.). *Why are some people healthy and others not? The determinants of health of populations*. New York: Aldine de Gruyter.

Fennema, M. 2004. "The Concept and Measurement of Ethnic Community." *Journal of Ethnic and Migration Studies*. Vol. 30. No. 3. pp. 429-447.

Fink, S. 2002. "International Efforts Spotlight Traditional, Complementary, and Alternative Medicine." *American Journal of Public Health*. Vol. 92. No. 10. pp. 1734-1739.

Fong, E. & R. Wilkes. 2003. "Racial and Ethnic Residential Patterns in Canada." *Sociological Forum*. Vol. 18. No. 4. pp. 577-602.

Hawe, P. & A. Shiell. 2000. "Social Capital and Health Promotion: A Review." *Social Science & Medicine*. Vol. 51. pp. 871-885.

Hedley, RA. 1980. "Work Values: A Test of the Convergence and Cultural Diversity Theses." *International Journal of Comparative Sociology*. Vol. 21. pp. 100-109.

Hellman, C.G. 1991. "Limits of the biomedical explanation." *Lancet*. Vol. 337. No. 8749. pp. 1080-1083.

Hudspith, M. 2005. "Barriers to Access to Care for Ethnic Minority Seniors." Unpublished notes.

Hufford, D. 2002. 'CAM and Cultural Diversity: Ethics and Epistemology Converge.' D. Callahan. (ed). in *The Role of Complementary and Alternative Medicine: Accommodating Pluralism*. Washington: Georgetown University Press.

Hufford, D. 1995. "Cultural and social perspectives on alternative medicine: background and assumptions." *Alternative Therapies in Health & Medicine*. Vol. 1. No. 2. pp. 53-62.

Inhorn, MC. & KL. Whittle. 2001. "Feminism meets the 'new' epidemiologies: toward an appraisal of antifeminist biases in epidemiological research on women's health." *Social Science & Medicine*. Vol. 53. pp. 553-567.

Kakai, H., Maskarinec, G., Shumay, D., Tatsumura, Y., & K Tasaki. 2003. "Ethnic differences in choices of health information by cancer patients using complementary and alternative medicine: an exploratory study with correspondence analysis." *Social Science & Medicine*. Vol. 56. pp. 851-862.

Kaptchuk, T. 2000. *The Web That Has No Weaver: Understanding Chinese Medicine*. New York: Contemporary Books.

Kelner, M. & B. Wellman. 1997. "Health care and consumer choice: Medical and alternative therapies." *Social Science & Medicine*. Vol. 45. No. 2. pp. 203-212.

Kobayashi, K.M. 2003. "Do Intersections of Diversity Matter? An Exploration of the Relationship Between Identity Markers and Health for Mid-to Later-life Canadians." *Canadian Ethnic Studies*. Vol. 35. No. 3. pp. 85-98.

Lee, M., Chang, J., Jacobs, B., & M. Wrensch. 2002. "Complementary and Alternative Medicine Use Among Men With Prostate Cancer in 4 Ethnic Populations." *American Journal of Public Health.* Vol. 92. No. 10. pp. 1606-1609.

Lee, R., Rodin, G., Devins, G., & M. Weiss. 2001. "Illness experience, meaning, and help-seeking among Chinese immigrants in Canada with chronic fatigue and weakness." *Anthropology & Medicine.* Vol. 8. No. 1. pp. 89-107.

Li, P. 2004. "Social Capital and Economic Outcomes for Immigrants and Ethnic Minorities." *Journal of International Migration and Integration.* Vol. 5. No. 2. pp. 171-190.

Ma, G.X. 1999. "Between Two Worlds: The Use of Traditional and Western Health Services by Chinese Immigrants." *Journal of Community Health.* Vol. 24. No. 6. pp. 421-437.

Maciocia, G. 1989. *The Foundations of Chinese Medicine.* Edinburgh: Churchill Livingstone.

Mackenzie, E., Taylor, L., Bloom, B., Hufford, D., & J. Johnson, 2003. "Ethnic minority use of complementary and alternative medicine (CAM): A national probability survey of CAM utilizers." *Alternative Therapies in Health and Medicine.* Vol. 9. No. 4. pp. 50-56.

McDonough P. & V. Walters. 2001. "Gender and health: reassessing patterns and explanations." *Social Science & Medicine.* Vol. 52. pp. 547-559.

McFarland, B., Bigelow, D., Zani, B., Newsom, J., & M. Kaplan. 2002. "Complementary and alternative medicine use in Canada and the United States." *American Journal of Public Health.* Vol. 92, No. 10. pp. 1616-1618.

McKinlay, JB. (1994). "A Case for Refocusing Upstream: The Political Economy of Illness."

Mishler, EG. 1981. "Viewpoint: Critical perspectives on the biomedical model." Pp. 1-23 in E. Mishler (Ed.), *Social Contexts of Health, Illness, and Patient Care.* Cambridge, UK: Cambridge University Press.

Millar, W. 1997. "Use of Alternative Health Care Practitioners by Canadians." *Canadian Journal of Public Health.* Vol. 88. No. 3. pp. 154-158.

Muntaner, C., Lynch, J. & G. Oates. 2001. "The social class determinants of income inequality and social cohesion." pp. 367-399 in V. Navarro (ed.). *Political Economy of Social Inequalities: Consequences for Health and Quality of Life.*

Nagel, J. 1994. "Constructing Ethnicity: Creating and Recreating Ethnic Identity and Culture." *Social Problems.* Vol 41. No. 1. pp. 152-176.

Najm, W., Reinsch, S., Hoehler, F., & J. Tobis. 2003. "Use of complementary and alternative medicine among the ethnic elderly." *Alternative Therapies in Health and Medicine*. Vol. 9. No. 3. pp. 50-57.

Navarro, V. & L. Shi. 2001. "The political context of social inequalities and health." *Social Science & Medicine*. Vol. 52. pp. 481-491.

Ou, B., Huang, D., Hampsch-Woodill, M., & J. Flanagan. 2003. "When East Meets West: The Relationship Between Yin-Yang and Antioxidation-Oxidation." *The Faseb Journal*. Vol. 17. pp. 127-129.

Pourat, N., Lubben, J., Wallace, S., & A. Moon. 1999. "Predictors of use of traditional Korean healers among elderly Koreans in Los Angeles." *The Gerontologist*. Vol. 39. No. 6. pp.710-719.

Robbins, K. 2005. "The origins, early development and status of Bourdieu's concept of 'cultural capital'." *The British Journal of Sociology*. Vol. 56. No. 3. pp. 13-30.

Saks, M. 2000. "Professionalization, Politics, and CAM." Pp.223-238 in Kelner et al., (eds.). *Complementary and Alternative Medicine: Challenge and Change*. Amsterdam: Harwood Academic Publishers.

Salaff, J., Fong, E. & Wong, S. 1999. "Using Social Networks to Exit Hong Kong." pp. 299-329 in Wellman, B. (ed). *Networks in the Global Village: Life in Contemporary Communities*. Boulder: Westview.

Salant, T. & D. Lauderdale. 2003. "Measuring Culture: A Critical Review of Acculturation and Health in Asian Immigrant Populations." *Social Science & Medicine*. Vol. 51. No. 1. pp. 71-90.

Satia-Abouta, J., Patterson, R., Kristal, A., Teh, C. & S. Tu. 2002. "Psychosocial Predictors of Diet and Acculturation in Chinese American and Chinese Canadian Women." *Ethnicity and Health*. Vol. 7. No. 1. pp. 21-39.

Schuller, T., Baron, S., & J. Field. 2000. "Social Captial: A Review and Critique." Pp. 1-38 in S. Baron et al. (eds.). *Social Capital: Critical Perspectives*. Oxford, UK: Oxford University Press.

Segall, A. & N. Chappell. 2000. *Health and Health Care in Canada*. Toronto, ON: Pearson Education Canada.

Statistics Canada, 2008. *A Portrait of the foreign-born population, 2006 Census*. Available from: http://www12.statcan.ca/census-recensement/2006/as-sa/ 97-557/p1-eng.cfm

Statistics Canada, 2008. *Ethnocultural Portrait of Canada*. Available from: http://www12.statcan.ca/english/census06/data/highlights/ethnic/index.cfm?Lang=E

Statistics Canada, 2005. "Canadian Community Health Survey (2003): User Guide for the Public Use Microdata File. Available at: http://www.statcan. ca/cgi-bin/imdb/p2SV.pl?Function=getSurvey&SDDS=3226&lang =en&db =IMDB&dbg=f&adm=8&dis=2

Struthers, R. & L. Nichols. 2004. "Utilization of complementary and alternative medicine among racial and ethnic minority populations: Implications for reducing health disparities." *Annual Review of Nursing.* Vol. 22. pp. 285-313.

Suzuki, N. 2004. "Complementary and Alternative Medicine: a Japanese Perspective." *ECam,* Vol. 1, No. 2. pp. 113-118.

Thorne, S. 1993. "Health belief systems in perspective." *Journal of Advanced Nursing.* Vol. 18. Pp. 1931-1931.

Ward, P. 2002. *White Canada Forever.* Montreal: McGill-Queen's University Press.

Waxler-Morrison, N. 2002. Personal Communication with Karen Kobayashi.

White, M.J., Fong, E., & Q. Cai. 2003. "The Segregation of Asian-Origin Groups in the United States and Canada." *Social Science Research.* Vol. 32. pp. 148-167.

Wilson, K. & A. Portes. 1980. "Immigrant Enclaves: An Analysis of the labor Market Experiences of Cubans in Miami." *American Journal of Sociology.* Vol. 86. pp. 295-319.

World Health Organization. 2010. "WHO definition of Health." Available from: http://www.who.int/about/definition/en/print.html/

Zhang, J. & M. Verhoef. 2002. "Illness Management Strategies among Chinese Immigrants Living with Arthritis." *Social Science and Medicine.* Vol. 55. No. 10. pp. 1795-1802.

Index